Contents

What Is the Ornish Diet?

The Ornish diet is designed to be a heart-healthy eating plan. It not only restricts dietary fat quite severely (to less than 10% of daily calories) but also requires that any ingested fats come from purely plant sources. In both the medical literature and in the popular press, the Ornish diet has been lauded as effective in preventing the progression of coronary artery disease (CAD) and even in facilitating an actual improvement in coronary artery plaques.

However, the idea that low-fat diets, such as those recommended for so many years by the U.S. government and the American Heart Association (AHA), are effective at preventing atherosclerotic cardiovascular disease has now been generally discredited. Over the past several decades, clinical studies in which dietary fat was restricted to less than 25% of daily calories have failed to demonstrate a cardiovascular benefit. Eventually, the AHA quietly dropped its low-fat diet recommendation.

How To Follow The Ornish Diet?

To follow the Ornish Diet:

• Eat all the beans, legumes, fruits, grains, and vegetables you need to feel full.

• Eat dairy low- or nonfat dairy products such as milk, cheese, and yogurt in moderation. Only 10 percent of your calories should come from fat.

• Avoid meats (red and white), oils and products containing oils, including avocados, olives, nuts, seeds, full-fat dairy, and sugar.

- Exercise for at least 30 minutes five times a week or 60 minutes three times a week.

- Manage stress with yoga and meditation and by spending time with your loved ones.

- Kick unhealthy habits such as smoking or drinking alcohol in excess.

- Eat smaller meals more often to combat hunger, but be careful not to overeat because you're eating more often.

u less likely to overeat out of frustration or anger.

Is Ornish Diet a heart-healthy diet?

Without question, the Ornish Diet is great for your heart. Ornish and a team of researchers were the first to show that heart disease, beyond being stoppable, can also be reversed, without drugs or surgery, through changes in diet and lifestyle. In a randomized trial of 48 heart-disease patients published in 1990 in The Lancet, the Ornish program to reverse heart disease reversed artery blockages after one year – and continued to do so after five years. The changes were highly meaningful when compared to a control group, whose condition worsened at both points. The diet has also been shown to lower blood pressure and decrease both total and bad LDL cholesterol.

Can Ornish Diet prevent or control diabetes?

The Ornish Diet can very likely prevent or control diabetes.

Prevention: Being overweight is one of the biggest risk factors for Type 2 diabetes. If you need to lose weight and keep it off, and an Ornish diet helps you do it, you'll almost certainly tilt the odds in your favor.

Control: Because you develop your own plan on the Ornish diet, you can ensure that what you're eating doesn't conflict with your doctor's advice. Ornish's basic principles of emphasizing whole grains and produce and shunning saturated fat and cholesterol are right in line with American Diabetes Association guidelines.

In the American Journal of Health Promotion analysis cited in the weight-loss section, 329 Ornish dieters decreased their hemoglobin A1C levels – a measure of blood sugar control – by

0.4 percentage points after a year. That was considered meaningful.

Is Ornish Diet nutritious?

Provided that you obey the limitations on what Dr. Dean Ornish calls group five foods heavy on saturated fat and instead stick with groups one through three at the other end of his spectrum – fish, plants, whole grains – your menu will stay in line with the federal government's recommendations and you won't risk your health.

Here's a breakdown of the nutritional content of a day's meals on two Ornish plans, alongside recommendations from the federal government's 2015-20 Dietary Guidelines for Americans.

Because this diet is highly individualized, your actual intake will vary. The first column reflects a dieter who chooses foods from the first three groups of Ornish's nutrition spectrum. The second is for a dieter on the plan to reverse heart disease. Diet figures were supplied by Ornish.

How It Works

The Ornish diet is a very low-fat vegetarian eating plan. Actually, it is a spectrum: On the more extreme end is the "reversal" program, used with the goal of reversing heart disease. A less-restrictive version is the "prevention" program. The Ornish diet also encompasses lifestyle changes including exercise, stress management (through breathing, meditation, and/or yoga), relationships (spending time with, and getting support from, loved ones), and smoking cessation, if you are a smoker.

What to Eat

Compliant Foods

- Fruits

- Vegetables

- Whole grains

- Legumes, seeds, and nuts

Non-Compliant Foods

- Meat, poultry, and fish

- Egg yolks

- Refined carbohydrates

- Saturated fats

- Dairy products (in excess)

- Alcohol and caffeine (in excess)

Fruits and Vegetables

This diet is vegetarian, so prepare for plenty of produce. In addition to those fruits and veggies, you will use vegetarian sources of fats, such as olive oil, for cooking.

Whole Grains

On this diet, you must swap refined carbohydrates for whole grain versions—so, whole-wheat bread instead of white, for example.

Legumes, Seeds, and Nuts

Legumes are a good source of protein in a plant-based diet. More nuts and seeds are available on the prevention plan.

Meat, Poultry, and Fish

On the reversal Ornish diet, no animal proteins are allowed, since they contain saturated fats. On the prevention plan, some fish is included since it is a good source of omega-3 fatty acids.

Eggs

Egg whites are permitted, but not yolks, because of their cholesterol content.

Dairy Products

Small amounts of nonfat milk or yogurt are allowed.

Modifications

The Ornish diet is not a singular plan, but a spectrum of offerings that range from very low-fat and completely vegetarian to more flexible options that incorporate fish, chicken, avocados, nuts, and seeds.

Pros and Cons

Pros

- No associated health risks

- Satisfies hunger

- Accessible

Cons

- Restrictive

- Hard to sustain

- Time-consuming

Pros

Safety

There are no special health risks associated with the Ornish diet, as long as basic nutritional needs (for protein, carbohydrates, and nutrients) are met. However, its health claims may not be completely supported by scientific evidence.

Satiety

Although the Ornish diet limits the types of foods that are consumed, it does not limit the amounts. Eating plenty of fruits, vegetables and whole grains can usually satisfy hunger.

Accessibility

No specialty foods are required on this diet, and the complaint foods are readily available.

Sometimes they can be more expensive (e.g., quinoa pasta vs. traditional versions), but you also save money by cutting out meat. In addition, there is no calorie-counting or food-tracking, which may be appealing to some users.

While there are many positive aspects of this diet, it is not a cure-all and it is not perfect for everyone.

Cons

Restrictiveness

Eating a low-fat, vegetarian diet still allows for balanced nutritional intake, as long as special attention is paid to iron and omega-3 fatty acids. However, cutting fat down to 10% of daily intake is challenging for most people. Due to protein limitations, this may lead to a higher carbohydrate intake which may not be beneficial for someone who has pre-diabetes or diabetes.

Sustainability

For that reason (the restriction on fats, not to mention refined carbs, alcohol, and caffeine), some people may find it difficult to follow this diet for the long term. It is meant to be a lifelong change, not a temporary one.

Time commitment

Eating vegetarian can take a lot of prep and cooking time. You also may need to learn how to cook differently, without meat and saturated fats. Also, most convenience foods and meals are off-limits on this diet.

How It Compares

The Ornish diet shares many characteristics with other low- or no-meat and "heart-healthy" diets. It also generally meets USDA recommendations on nutritional balance, with some planning and effort.

Calories

The USDA suggests roughly 2000 calories per day for weight maintenance, although this number can vary significantly based on age, sex, current weight, and activity level. The Ornish diet is based on reducing fat, not calories, so calorie intake will be different for everyone following the diet.

Similar Diets

This is how the Ornish diet compares to other low- or no-animal fat diets.

Ornish Diet

• Accessibility: No special foods, supplements, food tracking, or calorie counting are required.

• Effectiveness: Some studies have shown the Ornish diet can be effective in measures of heart health and weight loss.

• Sustainability: It may take some time to adjust to this style of eating, especially the "reversal" program. The prevention program is likely to be easier to follow and to stick with long term.

Vegetarian Diet

• Accessibility: Again, on a vegetarian diet, no special foods are required (unless you want meatless versions of foods like hot dogs or chicken tenders) and there's no tracking your food. Just avoid meats.

• Effectiveness: If you are going vegetarian to lose weight, you will still need to be aware of your calorie intake.

• Sustainability: Many people adapt to and enjoy a meat-free diet for life.

Vegan Diet

• Accessibility: People on a vegan diet do not consume any meat products at all, unlike vegetarians who do eat eggs and dairy products. It is more challenging to meet nutritional needs this way, and some special foods and supplements might be necessary.

- Effectiveness: Many people lose weight on a vegan diet, and there may be other heart-health and disease-prevention benefits.

- Sustainability: Like the Ornish diet, a vegan diet requires a significant commitment to sustain.

Mediterranean Diet

- Accessibility: The Mediterranean diet is probably the easiest to access. It does not eliminate meat, but de-emphasizes it in favor of fish, legumes, and some dairy products. It is not a low-fat diet.

- Effectiveness: Some studies have shown the Mediterranean diet to be more effective than lower-fat diets in weight loss and other health measures. The 2020 U.S. News and World

Report list of best diets ranks the Mediterranean diet as the #1 overall diet.

• Sustainability: The Mediterranean diet is meant to be a long-term lifestyle change, and that change is manageable for most people.

The Ornish Diet: Sample Menu

Here are two days of typical meals, both between 1,800 and 1,900 calories. The first menu is based on foods from Ornish's three healthiest food groups (out of five he divides foods into); the second is his plan to reverse heart disease. You can find recipes for these meals on the Ornish website.

Spectrum prevention plan

Breakfast

2 egg-white vegetable scramble.

1/3 cup each blueberries, strawberries and raspberries.

1/2 cup nonfat milk.

1 slice whole-grain bread.

Lunch

1 1/4 cup roasted-tomato soup

2 1/2 cups Asian noodle salad topped with 5 grilled shrimp

1 slice whole-wheat peach griddle cake

Snack

2/3 ounces dark chocolate

3 apricots

10 raw almonds

1/2 cup plain nonfat yogurt

Dinner

3-ounce wild salmon

1 1/4 cup butter lettuce/pear salad with honey-infused vinaigrette

1 1/2 cup sweet corn, black bean and tomato salad

5/8 cup peach bread pudding

Glass of wine or sparkling water

Spectrum reversing-heart-disease plan

Breakfast

1 3/4 egg-white zucchini frittata

1/3 cup each blueberries, strawberries and blackberries

1/2 cup nonfat milk

1 slice whole-grain bread

1 cup tea or decaf coffee

Lunch

1 7/8 cup mango-beet salad

1 7/8 cup vegetarian chili

1 slice corn bread

Snack

5/8 cup green pea guacamole

6 whole-wheat pita bread wedges

1/2 cup red grapes

Dinner

1 7/8 cup fennel and arugula salad with fig vinaigrette

2 cups whole-wheat penne pasta with roasted vegetables

2 1/3 cup fruit-and-yogurt trifle

Glass of wine or sparkling water

ORNISH DIET RECIPES

Trying new ornish-friendly recipes is a great way to explore new flavors and find new favorite dishes while looking after your health. In this part are nourishing ornish diet recipes for you to enjoy.

DEAN ORNISH'S GRANOLA

Preparation time

2 hours

INGREDIENTS

- 2 cups rolled oats

- 1/4 cup oat bran

- 1/2 cup rye flakes

- 2 tablespoons soy crumbles, See NOTE

- 1/4 cup apple juice

- 1 teaspoon vanilla

- 1 teaspoon ground cinnamon

- 1/2 teaspoon fresh grated nutmeg

- 1/4 cup dates, chopped and pitted

- 1/4 cup raisins

Instructions

1. Mix everything but the dates and raisins and toss to cover with the apple juice.

2. Bake for 1 1/2 to 2 hours at 300°F

3. Cool; add dates and raisins.

4. Place in airtight containers in a cool place

1-2-3 Tasty Morning Scramble

Preparation time

10 minutes

Ingredients

- 2 large egg whites beaten

- 1 pinch granulated garlic

- 1 bunch baby spinach

- 1/4 c chopped tomato

- 1 pinch fresh pepper

Instructions

1. Spray a non-stick pan with non-stick cooking spray.

2. Add spinach.

3. After spinach begins to wilt add eggs, garlic and salt and pepper.

4. Continue stirring the eggs until cooked.

5. Top with tomato.

Un-Do It Tacos

Preparation time

30 minutes

INGREDIENTS

- 6 corn tortillas

- 1 cup onion diced to ¼ inch

- 1 cup yellow corn fresh or frozen

- 1 cup water

- 1 envelope spicy taco seasoning mix, suggested brand: "Simply Organic" Southwest Taco

- 12 ounce package ground veggie crumbles, suggested brand: "Yves" MEXICAN SLAW (optional)

- 3 cups green cabbage finely sliced

- 3 cups purple cabbage finely sliced

- 12 ounce package silken tofu

- ¾ cup picante sauce mild, suggested brand: Pace

- 1/4 teaspoon salt (optional)

- Garnish (optional):

- Fat free cheddar cheese grated, suggested brand: LifeTime

- Chopped cilantro

INSTRUCTIONS

1. Simmer the onion, corn, water and seasoning mix together, in a pan over medium heat, until the onions are translucent.

2. Add and mix in the Veggie

3. Ground and cook the taco filling for a few minutes, stirring frequently for no more than 5 minutes.

4. While the taco filling is cooking, prepare the Mexican slaw.

5. Blend the tofu and the picante sauce in a blender or food processor and mix this dressing with the thinly sliced cabbage.

6. Heat the tortillas and serve them with the taco filling, the Mexican slaw, (optional) nonfat cheddar cheese and cilantro.

Ornish Apple Spice

Preparation time

45 minutes

INGREDIENTS

• Nonstick cooking spray

• 2 CUPS whole wheat flour or gluten-free flour
blend

• ½ CUP old-fashioned rolled oats

• ½ CUP flax meal

• 2 TEASPOONS pumpkin pie spice (see Chef's
Note)

- 1 TEASPOON baking powder

- 1 TEASPOON baking soda

- ½ TEASPOON fine sea salt

- ½ TEASPOON stevia powder

- 1 ¼ CUPS unsweetened applesauce

- ½ CUP apricot fruit spread (fruit juice-sweetened only)

- 1 CUP apple grated about 1 medium apple

- 1 CUP chopped dried apple

- ½ CUP raisins

- 2 TEASPOONS vanilla extract

Instructions

1. Preheat oven to 350ºF.

2. Spray a 12-cup non-stick muffin pan lightly with cooking spray, or line muffin pan with paper liners and spray liners lightly with cooking spray.

3. In a medium bowl, whisk together whole wheat flour or gluten-free flour blend, oatmeal, flax meal, pumpkin pie spice, baking powder, baking soda, salt, and stevia powder.

4. In a large bowl, stir together the applesauce, apricot fruit spread, grated apple, dried apple, raisins, and vanilla extract.

5. Stir in half the dry ingredients, then stir in the remaining half until just mixed.

6. The mixture may look lumpy.

7. Spoon one-third cup batter into each muffin cup.

8. Bake the muffins until a toothpick comes out clean from the center of a muffin, about 35 minutes. Be careful not to overcook.

9. Place muffin pan on a rack and let cool for 10 minutes, until muffins pull away slightly from the edges of the muffin cups.

10. Remove muffins from pan. Serve warm or let cool on a rack to room temperature.

Ornish Breakfast Quinoa Recipe

Preparation time

20 minutes

INGREDIENTS

For Quinoa:

- 1 CUP white quinoa

- 2 CUPS water

- 1/3 CUP golden or dark raisins

- PINCH fine sea salt

For Porridge:

- 1 ½ CUPS unsweetened soy milk

- 2 TEASPOONS vanilla extract

- ½ TEASPOON powdered stevia (optional)

- ½ TEASPOON pumpkin pie spice or cinnamon (see Chef's Note)

- PINCH fine sea salt

Instructions

1. 1. Using a fine-mesh strainer, rinse quinoa well.

2. 2. In a small 1½ quart heavy-bottomed saucepan, combine quinoa, water, raisins, and pinch of salt.

3. Over high heat, bring to a boil.

4. 3. Reduce heat to a simmer, cover, and cook until all water is absorbed, about 10 to 15 minutes.

5. 4. While quinoa is cooking, whisk together the soy milk, vanilla, stevia if using, pumpkin pie spice or cinnamon, and a pinch of salt in a medium bowl.

6. 5. Stir soy milk mixture into the quinoa.

7. Let simmer, stirring occasionally, until mixture is heated through, 1–2 minutes.

8. Divide into 6 bowls.

9. Sprinkle with additional pumpkin pie spice or cinnamon.

10. Serve warm.

Ornish Carrot Cupcakes with Non-fat Maple frosting

Preparation time

1 hour 5 minutes

INGREDIENTS

For Cupcakes:

- Nonstick cooking spray

- 2 ¼ CUPS whole-wheat pastry flour

- 1/3 CUP brown sugar

- 2 TEASPOONS baking powder

- 1 TEASPOON powdered stevia

- 1 ½ TEASPOONS cinnamon

- ¾ TEASPOON fine sea salt

- ¼ TEASPOON nutmeg

- 1/8 TEASPOON ground cloves

- 1 TABLESPOON ground flax meal

- 1 TABLESPOON water

- 1 ½ CUPS carrot grated, 3 medium carrots

- ¾ CUP unsweetened almond milk

- ½ CUP unsweetened applesauce

- 2 TEASPOONS vanilla extract

For Frosting:

- ONE 8-OZ PACKAGE nonfat cream cheese at room temperature

- 1/3 CUP pure maple syrup

- 1 TEASPOON vanilla extract

Instructions

1. Preheat oven to 375ºF. Lightly spray a muffin pan with nonstick cooking spray, or line cups with paper liners and lightly spray liners.

2. In a large bowl, mix together whole wheat pastry flour, brown sugar, baking powder, stevia, cinnamon, salt, nutmeg, and cloves.

3. In a medium bowl, mix flax meal with water. Let sit until water is absorbed, 1 to 2 minutes.

Add carrots, almond milk, applesauce, and vanilla extract.

4. Stir the carrot mixture into the flour mixture. Mix well.

5. Spoon 1/4 cup batter into each muffin cup.

6. Bake for 30 to 35 minutes, until a toothpick inserted in the center comes out clean.

7. Remove from oven and let cool on a rack.

8. Place muffin pan on a rack and let cupcakes cool in the pan for 10 minutes, until cupcakes pull away slightly from the edges of the muffin cups.

9. Remove cupcakes from pan and let cool completely on a rack. Cupcakes should be completely cool before frosting.

10. To make the frosting, in a small bowl, combine cream cheese, maple syrup, and vanilla extract.

11. Using a hand-held electric mixer, beat on high speed until smooth.

12. To frost cupcakes, spread a heaping tablespoon of frosting evenly across the top of each cupcake just before serving. These are best enjoyed the day they are made.

Ornish Cocoa Truffles

Preparation time

15 minutes

INGREDIENTS

- 1 CUP FRESH pitted medjool dates firmly packed about 9 dates, or 6 oz

- ½ CUP unsweetened cocoa powder (suggested brand: Hershey or Green & Black 100% cacao powder)

- 1 ½ TEASPOONS vanilla extract

- ¼ TEASPOON fine sea salt

- ½ TEASPOON cinnamon (optional: for Mexican Truffles)

- 1/8 TEASPOON cayenne pepper (optional: for Mexican Truffle)

- ¼ CUP unsweetened cocoa powder (optional: for rolling)

- ¼ CUP turbinado (raw) sugar (optional: for rolling)

Instructions

1. Place dates in a small bowl.

2. Cover with hot water and let soak for 15 minutes. Drain and pat dry.

3. Using a food processor fitted with a metal blade, pulse dates several times to make a paste. Add cocoa powder, vanilla, and salt.

4. To make Mexican Truffles, add cinnamon and cayenne. Pulse 3 or 4 times (mixture will seem dry).

5. Add 1 tablespoon warm water, and pulse several more times, adding another tablespoon of warm water if mixture still seems dry.

6. Continue to pulse until mixture is smooth and forms a ball.

7. Remove truffle mixture from processor and transfer to a bowl.

8. Put ¼ cup cocoa powder or turbinado (raw) sugar in a shallow bowl. Using 1 tablespoon of truffle mixture for each ball, shape balls between the palms of your hands. (If mixture seems sticky, refrigerate until well chilled before rolling.) Roll each ball in cocoa powder or sugar after shaping.

9. Cover and refrigerate until serving.

Ornish Egg White and Vegetable Frittata

Preparation time

40 minutes

INGREDIENTS

- 2 CUPS white mushrooms thinly sliced

- 4 oz

- 1 CUP zucchini coarsely chopped

- 1 CUP yellow onion diced

- ½ CUP dried tomatoes cut into thin strips

- 1 TABLESPOON fresh thyme, divided chopped

- 2 TEASPOONS garlic pressed or minced

- ½ TEASPOON fine sea salt

- ½ TEASPOON freshly ground pepper, divided

- ½ CUP water

- 2 CUPS kale finely chopped

- 2 CUPS egg whites (from 18 eggs) or 16 oz prepared liquid egg whites

- 3 TABLESPOONS nutritional yeast

- 1 ½ TEASPOONS Better than Bouillon No-Chicken Base

- 1 ½ TEASPOONS sweet rice flour or cornstarch

- ½ TEASPOON onion powder

- Nonstick spray (optional)

- ½ TEASPOON paprika for garnish

- ½ CUP cherry tomatoes halved for garnish

Instructions

1. Preheat oven to 350ºF.

2. In a large, heavy-bottomed saute pan over medium heat, combine mushrooms, zucchini, yellow onion, dried tomatoes, 2 teaspoons of the thyme, garlic, salt, and 1/4 teaspoon of the pepper with ½ cup water.

3. Cook, stirring frequently, until vegetables are soft and onions are translucent, 8–10 minutes.

4. Add kale. Cook, stirring frequently, until kale is tender, about 5 minutes. Add up to 2 more tablespoons water if necessary, if vegetables seem dry or are starting to brown. Any extra

water should evaporate by the time the kale is tender.

5. In a blender, combine egg whites, nutritional yeast, bouillon base, sweet rice flour or cornstarch, onion powder, remaining teaspoon of thyme and ¼ teaspoon of pepper.

6. Blend at medium speed for 10 seconds, until ingredients are well mixed.

7. Lightly spray an 8 x 8-in glass baking pan with nonstick spray, or use a nonstick baking pan.

8. Spread vegetables evenly over bottom of baking pan. Pour egg mixture evenly over vegetables.

9. Sprinkle lightly with paprika.

10. Cover pan with aluminum foil.

11. Bake frittata for 20 minutes. Remove foil and continue to bake until frittata is set in the middle and edges are lightly browned, about 10 to 15 minutes. Remove frittata from the oven.

12. Let sit for at least 10 minutes before serving.

13. Cut frittata into four 4 x 4-in squares. Garnish each square with tomato halves.

Ornish Apple Spice Muffins

Preparation time

45 minutes

INGREDIENTS

Nonstick cooking spray

• 2 CUPS whole wheat flour or gluten-free flour blend

• ½ CUP old-fashioned rolled oats

• ½ CUP flax meal

• 2 TEASPOONS pumpkin pie spice (see Chef's Note)

• 1 TEASPOON baking powder

• 1 TEASPOON baking soda

• ½ TEASPOON fine sea salt

• ½ TEASPOON stevia powder

• 1 ¼ CUPS unsweetened applesauce

• ½ CUP apricot fruit spread (fruit juice-sweetened only)

- 1 CUP apple grated about 1 medium apple

- 1 CUP chopped dried apple

- ½ CUP raisins

- 2 TEASPOONS vanilla extract

Instructions

1. Preheat oven to 350ºF.

2. Spray a 12-cup non-stick muffin pan lightly with cooking spray, or line muffin pan with paper liners and spray liners lightly with cooking spray.

3. In a medium bowl, whisk together whole wheat flour or gluten-free flour blend, oatmeal, flax meal, pumpkin pie spice, baking powder, baking soda, salt, and stevia powder.

4. In a large bowl, stir together the applesauce, apricot fruit spread, grated apple, dried apple, raisins, and vanilla extract.

5. Stir in half the dry ingredients, then stir in the remaining half until just mixed. The mixture may look lumpy.

6. Spoon one-third cup batter into each muffin cup.

7. Bake the muffins until a toothpick comes out clean from the center of a muffin, about 35 minutes. Be careful not to overcook.

8. Place muffin pan on a rack and let cool for 10 minutes, until muffins pull away slightly from the edges of the muffin cups.

9. Remove muffins from pan. Serve warm or let cool on a rack to room temperature.

Ornish Caesar Salad

Preparation time

35 minutes

INGREDIENTS

For Dressing:

- 6 OZ silken tofu drained

- 2 TABLESPOONS water

- 2 TABLESPOONS fresh lemon juice

- 1 TABLESPOON red wine vinegar

- 1 TABLESPOON capers rinsed and drained (optional)

- 1 ½ TEASPOONS vegan Worcestershire sauce

- 1 ½ TEASPOONS prepared horseradish

- 1 TEASPOON garlic pressed or minced

- 2 TABLESPOONS nutritional yeast

- 1 TEASPOON dry mustard powder such as Coleman's

- ½ TEASPOON onion powder

- ¼ TEASPOON salt

- 1/8 TEASPOON freshly ground pepper

For Salad:

- 4 SLICES whole grain bread or 1 ½ cups packaged fat-free croutons

- 8 CUPS romaine lettuce torn or roughly chopped

- 2 carrots peeled and thinly sliced

- ½ CUP radishes thinly sliced

Instructions

1. To make the dressing, in a blender, combine tofu, water, lemon juice, red wine vinegar, capers, if using, Worcestershire sauce, horseradish, garlic, nutritional yeast, mustard powder, onion powder, salt, and pepper.

2. Blend on high speed for about 10 seconds, until mixture is smooth. (Dressing can be prepared several days in advance and refrigerated until needed.)

3. If making croutons, preheat oven to 250ºF. Line a baking sheet with parchment paper. Trim crusts from bread slices. Cut bread into 1-inch cubes (or preferred crouton size). Spread on prepared baking sheet. Bake until crisp throughout, about 15 to 20 minutes. Let cool.

4. In a large bowl, combine romaine lettuce, carrots, radishes and croutons, if using. Add half of the dressing. Toss and taste for seasoning. Add additional dressing as needed. Serve immediately.

Ornish Chocolate Pudding

Preparation time

5 minutes

INGREDIENTS

- 16 OZ firm silken tofu patted dry 2 cups

- ¾ CUP unsweetened cocoa powder (suggested brand: Hershey's)

- ¼ CUP pure maple syrup

- ¼ CUP water

- 1 TABLESPOON pure vanilla extract

- 1 ½ TEASPOONS powdered stevia

- PINCH fine sea salt

- 1 CUP raspberries or chopped strawberries garnish, optional

Instructions

1. In the bowl of a food processor fitted with a metal blade, combine tofu, cocoa powder, maple syrup, water, vanilla extract, stevia, and salt. Process until mixture is smooth and creamy, stopping as necessary to scrape down sides and center of the bowl with a rubber spatula.

2. Taste and adjust seasoning as needed with more maple syrup and/or vanilla.

3. Adjust consistency with a little more water as needed.

4. Divide pudding mixture between 6 small serving dishes. Refrigerate until chilled, about least 30 minutes.

5. Top each portion with berries, if using.

Ornish Edamole

Preparation time

10 minutes

INGREDIENTS

- 2 CUPS frozen shelled edamame thawed

- ¾ CUP silken tofu

- 1–2 CLOVES garlic pressed or minced to taste

- ½ TEASPOON ground cumin

- 2 TABLESPOONS fresh lime juice

- ½ –1 TEASPOON fine sea salt to taste

- ¼ TEASPOON lime zest (optional)

- 1 small tomato seeded and diced (optional)

- ¼ CUP cilantro chopped (optional)

- 2 TABLESPOONS red onion diced (optional)

- 2–3 DASHES hot sauce, green or red (optional)

Instructions

1. In a food processor, combine edamame, tofu, garlic, cumin, lime juice, and 1/2 teaspoon of the salt.

2. Pulse until ingredients are blended to desired texture; you can stop while mixture is still chunky and coarse or continue to process into a smooth, thick paste.

3. Use a rubber spatula to scrape down the sides as needed.

4. Transfer mixture to a bowl. Taste for seasoning and add additional salt as needed. Stir in lime zest, diced tomato, cilantro, red onion, and/or hot sauce, if using.

5. Serve as a dip with an assortment of raw vegetables and fat-free whole grain crackers, or use as a sandwich spread.

Ornish Eggplant Parmesan

Preparation time

2 hours

INGREDIENTS

For Eggplant:

• ½ CUP egg whites from 4 eggs

• ¼ TEASPOON fine sea salt

• 1 ¼ CUPS fat-free, whole-grain (or gluten-free) breadcrumbs

- 2 small to medium eggplants cut into 1/2-in slices (about 16 to 20 slices total) see Chef's Note

For Filling:

- 1 LB frozen spinach thawed

- 8 OZ firm tofu patted dry and finely crumbled

- ¾ TEASPOON garlic powder

- ¾ TEASPOON onion powder

- ¼ TEASPOON fine sea salt

- 1/8 TEASPOON freshly ground pepper

For Assembly:

- ONE 24-OZ jar low-fat marinara sauce

- 1 CUP fat-free mozzarella cheese shredded (optional)

- ¼ CUP fresh basil chopped

Instructions

1. Preheat oven to 375ºF. Line a baking sheet with parchment paper.

2. Place egg whites and ¼ teaspoon salt in a small, shallow bowl.

3. Whisk vigorously with a fork until light and frothy.

4. Place breadcrumbs in a second small shallow bowl.

5. One slice at a time, dip eggplant into the egg whites, coating each side.

6. Then, dip each slice into the breadcrumbs, coating each side.

7. Press the crumbs onto each slice as necessary to make them stick. (So your hands don't get gloppy, use one hand to dip the eggplant into the egg whites and the other to dip into the crumbs.)

8. Place crumb-coated eggplant slices on the prepared baking sheet.

9. Bake until eggplant slices are cooked through and lightly brown on top, about 35 minutes.

10. Remove the eggplant from the oven.

11. While eggplant is baking, make the filling.

12. Place thawed spinach in a colander in the sink or over a deep bowl.

13. Using your hands, squeeze or press spinach vigorously to remove excess liquid.

14. Continue to squeeze and press spinach until it is almost dry.

15. After draining, you should have about 1½ cups of spinach.

16. In a medium bowl, stir together the drained spinach, finely crumbled tofu, onion powder, garlic powder, 1/4 teaspoon salt and pepper. Set aside.

17. To assemble the eggplant parmesan, spread 1 cup of marinara sauce evenly over the bottom of a 9 x 13-in glass Pyrex baking dish. Arrange 8 to 10 of the baked eggplant slices on top of the marinara.

18. Spoon 1/3 cup of the spinach mixture on top of each piece of eggplant. Top each piece of eggplant with a heaping tablespoon of marinara sauce.

19. Top each eggplant slice with another, similarly-sized slice of eggplant, lightly pressing the slices together.

20. Spoon the remaining marinara sauce over the eggplant slices. Sprinkle slices with cheese, if using. (Recipe can be prepared up to this point, 1 to 2 days in advance. Cover and refrigerate until needed. Preheat oven to 375ºF before baking.)

21. Bake the eggplant parmesan until eggplant and filling have heated through and cheese has melted, 30–35 minutes.

22. To brown top, increase oven heat to broil. Move baking dish to the upper third of the oven, about 6 to 8 inches below the heat. Broil for one to two minutes, until the top is lightly browned and bubbly. Remove from the oven. Sprinkle with basil just before serving.

Ornish White Bean and Winter Green Soup

Preparation time

40 minutes

INGREDIENTS

- 1 ½ CUPS onion coarsely chopped

- 2 TEASPOONS garlic minced

- 4 CUPS low-sodium vegetable broth, divided

- 3 CUPS cooked cannellini or navy beans or two 15-oz cans cannellini or navy beans, rinsed and drained

- 2 CUPS sweet potatoes peeled and coarsely chopped

- 3 TABLESPOONS sweet white miso

- 2 TEASPOONS fresh thyme, divided chopped

- ¼ TEASPOON fine sea salt

- ¼ TEASPOON freshly ground pepper

- 2 CUPS FIRMLY PACKED kale or chard tough ribs removed, roughly chopped

- 1 ½ oz Crushed red pepper flakes (optional)

Instructions

1. In a 3-quart saucepan over medium heat, combine onion, garlic, and ½ cup of the broth.

2. Cook, stirring frequently, until onions are softened and transparent, about 10 minutes.

3. Add the remaining 3 1/2 cups of broth, beans, sweet potatoes, miso, 1 1/2 teaspoons of the thyme, salt and pepper.

4. Bring to a simmer and cook until sweet potatoes are tender and flavors have melded, about 10 to 15 minutes.

5. Add kale and remaining ½ teaspoon thyme.

6. Simmer until kale is tender, about 3 to 4 minutes.

7. Taste for seasoning, adding more miso or pepper as needed.

8. Sprinkle with crushed red pepper flakes before serving, if desired. This soup is best made one to two days in advance; cover and refrigerate until needed.

Ornish Lentil Loaf

Preparation time

2 hours

INGREDIENTS

- 1 CUP uncooked short grain brown rice

- 1 CUP uncooked French black or green lentils

- 8 OZ frozen spinach thawed

- 1 ½ CUPS onion diced

- 1 ½ CUPS carrots grated

- 1 TABLESPOON garlic pressed or minced

- 2 TABLESPOONS Bragg Liquid Aminos, divided

- 1 TABLESPOON fresh thyme, divided or 1 ½ teaspoons dried thyme, divided

- 1 TEASPOON dried oregano

- 1/2 TEASPOON freshly ground pepper, divided

- 1 CUP water, divided plus more as needed

- Smoky Chipotle Ketchup (see description, above, for recipe link)

Instructions

1. Preheat oven to 375ºF. Prepare rice and lentils according to package instructions. (The rice and lentils can be prepared up to two days ahead of time, and refrigerated until needed.)

2. Place thawed spinach in a colander in the sink or over a deep bowl. Using your hands, squeeze or press spinach vigorously to remove excess liquid. Continue to squeeze and press spinach until it is almost dry; excess liquid left in the spinach will make a soggy loaf. Once drained, you should have about ¾ cup of spinach. Set aside.

3. In a large saute pan over medium-low heat, sauté the onions, carrots, garlic, 1 tablespoon of the Bragg liquid aminos, 1 1/2 teaspoons of the fresh thyme, oregano, ¼ teaspoon of the

pepper, and ½ cup of the water. Stirring frequently, saute until onions are translucent, 7–10 minutes.

4. In a large bowl, combine the cooked rice and the lentils with the onion mixture. Add the remaining 1 tablespoon liquid aminos, 1 1/2 teaspoons fresh thyme and 1/4 teaspoon pepper. Mix well.

5. Spoon half of the rice mixture (about 3 1/2 cups) into a food processor. Pulse, adding ½ cup water as needed, until mixture is a thick paste. Mix this back into the remaining lentil mixture. Add the spinach and stir well to combine.

6. Line a baking sheet with parchment paper. Form and tightly pack lentil mixture into a loaf 2 inches high and 9 inches long. Bake for about 40

minutes, or until it is lightly browned and crisped on the top. Remove from oven and spread ½ cup Smoky Chipotle Ketchup evenly on top. Let cook for an additional 10 minutes. Remove from oven. (If you have an instant-read or digital thermometer, the internal temperature should read 165–170ºF.)

7. Let loaf rest for 10 minutes before slicing and serving.

Ornish Fast and Sloppy Joes

Preparation time

5 minutes

INGREDIENTS

- ONE 12-OZ PACKAGE vegetarian ground-meat alternative (suggested brand: Yves Veggie Ground or Lightlife Smart Ground)

- 1½ CUPS cooked pinto beans or one 15-oz can, rinsed and drained

- ½ CUP prepared barbecue sauce

- 1/3 CUP tomato paste

- 2/3 CUP water

- ¼ CUP green onions (scallions) chopped

- 2 TEASPOONS apple cider vinegar

- ½ TEASPOON smoked paprika

- ¼ TEASPOON freshly ground black pepper

- 6 whole-grain buns (less than 3 grams of fat, with 3 grams or more of fiber)

- ¾ CUP nonfat cheese, such as Monterey Jack or mozzarella shredded (optional)

- ¼ CUP green onions (scallions) chopped for garnish

Instructions

1. In a medium saucepan over medium heat, combine ground meat alternative, pinto beans, and barbecue sauce. In a small bowl, whisk together tomato paste and water until smooth. Add tomato paste to bean mixture along with ¼ cup green onions, apple cider vinegar, smoked paprika, and pepper.

2. Reduce heat to low and cook, stirring occasionally, until mixture is warm and flavors

have melded, 5-7 minutes. While filling is cooking, toast buns.

3. To serve as a closed sandwich, spoon ½ cup filling onto bottom half of bun. Top with 2 tablespoons grated nonfat cheese and a sprinkle of green onions, if using. Top with top half of bun. To serve open faced, spoon ¼ cup filling over each half of bun. Top each half with 1 tablespoon nonfat grated cheese and a sprinkle of green onion, if using.

Ornish White Bean and Carrot Soup

Preparation time

1 hour 15 minutes

INGREDIENTS

- 2 CUPS dry white beans such as Great Northern, cannellini, or navy

- 7 CUPS low-sodium vegetable broth

- 1 bay leaf

- 3 CUPS carrots peeled and diced

- 2 CUPS onions peeled and diced

- 1 TABLESPOON garlic pressed or minced

- 1 TABLESPOON fresh thyme chopped or 1 teaspoon dried

- 1 TABLESPOON fresh marjoram or oregano chopped or 1 teaspoon dried

- ¼ TEASPOON fine sea salt

- ¼ TEASPOON freshly ground pepper

Instructions

1. In a medium bowl, cover beans with cold water by several inches. Let soak for at least 8 hours or overnight.

2. Drain the soaked beans, discarding soaking liquid. In a large pot over high heat, combine beans with vegetable broth and bring to a boil.

3. Skim off any foam that forms on the surface.

4. Reduce heat to medium-low.

5. Add bay leaf. Partially cover and let simmer, stirring occasionally, for 15 minutes.

6. Add carrots, onions, garlic, thyme, marjoram, salt, and pepper. Let simmer, partially covered, until beans are tender, about 45 minutes. Remove from heat.

7. Remove bay leaf and discard.

8. Measure out 2 cups of the cooked beans along with ½ cup of the cooking liquid.

9. Place beans and cooking liquid in a blender. Blend until smooth, adding additional cooking liquid if necessary.

10. Return bean puree to the remaining beans and liquid in the pot and stir to combine.

11. Taste for seasoning, adding additional salt and/or pepper as needed. Reheat as necessary for serving.

Ornish Mac 'n Cheez

Preparation time

25 minutes

INGREDIENTS

For Sauce:

- 1 TABLESPOON arrowroot or cornstarch

- 1 TABLESPOON water

- 2 CUPS unsweetened soy milk

- ¼ CUP nutritional yeast plus more for garnish

- ¼ CUP white miso paste or white chickpea miso

- 2 TABLESPOONS tomato paste

- 2 TEASPOONS onion powder

- 1 TEASPOON dry mustard

For Pasta:

- ONE 8.8-OZ PACKAGE whole grain or gluten-free penne pasta, or preferred shape

- 4 CUPS broccoli florets (8 oz)

- 1/8 TEASPOON freshly ground pepper

- Paprika or smoked paprika for garnish

Instructions

1. Bring a large, heavy-bottomed pot of water to a boil.

2. In a small bowl, whisk arrowroot or cornstarch with 1 tablespoon water until dissolved.

3. In a small saucepan over medium heat, whisk together soy milk, nutritional yeast, white miso, tomato paste, onion powder, and dry mustard. Bring to a simmer.

4. Reduce heat to medium-low and whisk in arrowroot or cornstarch mixture. Cook, whisking frequently, until sauce thickens, 2–3 minutes. Cover and set aside to keep warm.

5. Cook pasta in pot of boiling water according to package instructions. Cook until pasta is cooked through but still firm to the bite ("al dente").

6. While pasta is cooking, place a vegetable steamer basket in a saucepan and add water to just below bottom of steamer basket. Over medium heat, bring water to a boil. Add broccoli. Cover and steam until broccoli is just tender but still bright green, 4 to 5 minutes.

7. Drain pasta and broccoli and return to the empty pasta pot. Add the warm sauce and toss to coat. Garnish with a sprinkle of paprika. Serve with additional nutritional yeast.

Ornish Traditional Split Pea Soup

Preparation time

1 hour

INGREDIENTS

- 2 CUPS split peas, green or yellow rinsed (12 oz)

- 8 CUPS water

- 2 CUPS red-skinned potatoes coarsely chopped (12 oz)

- 2 CUPS onion peeled and coarsely chopped

- 1 ½ CUPS carrots peeled and coarsely chopped

- 1 ½ CUPS celery coarsely chopped

- 2 TABLESPOONS garlic pressed or minced

- 1 TABLESPOON fresh oregano or 1 teaspoon dried

- 1 TABLESPOON fresh rosemary or 1 teaspoon dried

- 1 TABLESPOON fresh thyme or 1 teaspoon dried

- 1 ½ TEASPOONS Better than Bouillon No-Beef Base

- 1 TABLESPOON sherry vinegar

- ½ TEASPOON natural liquid smoke (optional)

- ½ TEASPOON fine sea salt

- ½ TEASPOON freshly ground pepper

Instructions

1.   In a large, heavy-bottomed pot over high heat, combine all ingredients and bring to a boil.

2.   Reduce heat to medium and simmer, stirring occasionally, until peas are very soft and vegetables are tender, 35–45 minutes.

3.   Taste for seasoning, adding additional vinegar, salt and/or pepper as needed.

Ornish Moroccan Vegetable Stew Recipe

Preparation time

1 hour 20 minutes

INGREDIENTS

- 2 CUPS onion peeled and diced

- 2 TEASPOONS garlic pressed or minced

- 1 ½ TABLESPOONS fresh ginger root peeled and finely chopped

- 2 TEASPOONS ground coriander, divided

- 1 cinnamon stick, about 3" long

- ½ TEASPOON turmeric

- ¼ TEASPOON fine sea salt

- 3 ½ CUPS low-sodium vegetable broth

- 3 CUPS butternut squash peeled and chopped (1 lb)

- ONE 14.5-OZ CAN fire-roasted diced tomatoes (suggested brand: Muir Glen)

- 2 CUPS green beans cut to 1-in lengths (½ lb)

- 1 ½ CUPS cooked garbanzo beans (chickpeas) or one 15-oz can, rinsed and drained

- ½ CUP golden raisins firmly packed

- ZEST OF 1 lemon

- ½ CUP cilantro chopped

- 1 ½ CUPS cooked quinoa warmed (FOR SERVING)

Instructions

1. In a large, 4 quart saucepan over medium heat, combine onions, garlic, ginger, 1 1/2 teaspoons of the coriander, cinnamon stick, turmeric, and salt with 1/2 cup of the vegetable broth.

2. Sauté, stirring frequently, for 7–10 minutes, until onions are softened and translucent.

3. Add remaining 3 cups vegetable broth, butternut squash, and tomatoes. Increase heat to high and bring to a boil.

4. Reduce heat to medium and simmer for about 30 minutes, until squash is just barely cooked through.

5. Add green beans, garbanzo beans, raisins, and lemon zest. Cook for 7–10 minutes, until green beans are tender.

6. Stir in remaining ½ teaspoon coriander.

7. Just before serving, stir in cilantro.

8. Serve warm, over quinoa.

Ornish Tofu Teryaki

Preparation time

50 minutes

INGREDIENTS

- 1 CUP unseasoned sake

- 1 CUP mirin (sweet rice wine)

- ¾ CUP water

- 1/3 CUP reduced-sodium tamari or soy sauce

- 1 TABLESPOON fresh ginger root peeled and finely chopped

- 1 TABLESPOON fresh garlic pressed or minced

- 1 ½ LB extra-firm tofu cut into ½ inch cubes (6 cups)

- 4 CUPS fresh shiitake, cremini, or white mushrooms, or a combination stems removed, quartered (1 lb)

- 1 CUP onion peeled and coarsely chopped

- 3 TABLESPOONS sweet rice flour or cornstarch

- ¼ CUP water

- 1 LARGE HEAD broccoli or 4 cups florets

- 1/3 CUP scallions thinly sliced (optional)

- 3 CUPS cooked brown rice (optional, for serving)

Instructions

1. Preheat oven to 350ºF. In a large bowl, combine sake, mirin, 3/4 cup water, tamari or

soy sauce, ginger and garlic. Add the tofu, stirring to coat. Marinate for at least 30 minutes. (Tofu can be marinated for several hours, or overnight.) After marinating, strain the tofu, reserving the marinade.

2. Line a baking sheet with parchment paper. Spread tofu cubes evenly over baking sheet. Bake until tofu is lightly browned, about 30 minutes. Remove from oven and set aside.

3. Place a steamer basket in a saucepan and add water to just below the bottom of steamer basket. Over high heat, bring water to a boil. Add broccoli florets. Cover and cook until broccoli is just tender, about 3 minutes. Remove basket and rinse broccoli quickly with cold water. Drain and set aside.

4. In a large, heavy-bottomed saute pan over medium-high heat, bring mushrooms, onions and 3/4 cup of the reserved tofu marinade to a simmer. Simmer, stirring frequently, until mushrooms are softened and onions are translucent, about 7–10 minutes.

5. Add remaining marinade, bring to a simmer and cook for 3 to 4 minutes to evaporate the alcohol from the mixture.

6. In a small bowl, whisk sweet rice flour or cornstarch with ¼ cup water until smooth. Whisk this mixture into the mushrooms and cook until glossy and thickened, 1–2 minutes. Add tofu, broccoli, and scallions, if using, reserving about 1 tablespoon of scallions for garnish. Cook,

stirring frequently until tofu and vegetables are heated through.

7. Serve over rice, if using. Garnish with reserved scallions.

Ornish Pasta Carbonara

Preparation time

30 minutes

Ingredients

• 6 OUNCES uncooked whole grain or gluten-free penne pasta (2 cups)

• 2/3 CUP frozen baby peas

• 2 CUPS broccoli florets (5 oz)

- ¼ CUP dried tomatoes not oil-packed

- 2 CUPS unsweetened low-fat soy milk

- ¼ CUP Roasted Garlic puree (see description, above, for link)

- 2 TABLESPOONS white miso

- 1 ½ TABLESPOONS nutritional yeast

- 1 ½ TEASPOONS fresh oregano finely chopped or ½ teaspoon dried

- 1 TEASPOON chipotle pepper in adobo sauce

- 1 TEASPOON sweet paprika

- 2 TEASPOONS arrowroot, cornstarch, or sweet rice flour

- 1 TABLESPOON water

- Fine sea salt to taste

• Freshly ground pepper to taste

Instructions

1. Fill a large saucepan two-thirds full of water.

2. Bring to boil over high heat.

3. Cook pasta according to package directions. One minute before pasta is ready, add peas.

4. Drain pasta and peas in a colander and set aside.

5. While pasta is cooking, place a vegetable steamer basket in a saucepan and add water to just below bottom of steamer basket. Over medium heat, bring water to a boil. Add broccoli.

6. Cover and steam until broccoli is just tender but still bright green, 4 to 5 minutes.

7. Remove basket from steamer and set aside.

8. In a small bowl, cover dried tomatoes with hot water.

9. Let stand until tomatoes are softened, about 5 minutes. Drain. Slice tomatoes into strips.

10. In a medium-sized, heavy-bottomed saucepan over medium heat, whisk together soy milk, roasted garlic, miso, nutritional yeast, oregano, chipotle pepper, and paprika. Add drained tomato and bring mixture to a simmer.

11. Cook, whisking frequently, until mixture starts to thicken, 4–5 minutes.

12. In a small bowl, whisk arrowroot with 1 tablespoon water to make a smooth paste. Whisk paste into sauce and cook until mixture thickens, 1–2 minutes.

13. Just before serving, stir pasta, peas, and broccoli into sauce. Cook, stirring, until mixture is heated through. Taste for seasoning, adding salt and/or pepper as needed. Serve immediately.

Ornish Spinach and Mushroom Egg White Scramble Recipe

Preparation time

20 minutes

INGREDIENTS

- 1 ½ CUPS onions diced

- 4 CUPS white mushrooms sliced

- ¼ CUP water

- ½ TEASPOON turmeric

- ½ TEASPOON garlic powder

- ¼ TEASPOON freshly ground pepper, divided

- 1/8 TEASPOON fine sea salt

- 1 ½ CUPS egg whites from approximately 8 eggs

- 4 CUPS baby spinach leaves

- Smoked paprika for garnish (optional)

Instructions

1. In a large 12-inch sauté pan over medium heat, combine onions, mushrooms, water,

turmeric, garlic powder, 1/8 teaspoon of the pepper, and salt.

2. Cook, stirring occasionally, until mushrooms are tender, onions are translucent, and all moisture has evaporated, about 7 to 10 minutes.

3. Add egg whites and remaining 1/8 teaspoon pepper.

4. Cook, stirring frequently, until egg whites are opaque.

5. Just before the egg whites are fully cooked, fold in the spinach. Continue cooking until spinach is wilted and any excess liquid has evaporated. Taste for seasoning, adding additional salt if desired.

6. Sprinkle with smoked paprika, if using. Serve immediately.

Ornish Reversal Hummus Recipe

Preparation time

5 minutes

INGREDIENTS

• 3 CUPS cooked garbanzo beans (chickpeas) or two 15-oz cans no salt added garbanzo beans, rinsed and drained

• ½ CUP water

• 1 ½ TABLESPOONS lemon juice

• 2 TEASPOONS ground cumin

• 1 ½ TEASPOONS ground coriander

- 1 TEASPOON garlic finely chopped or pressed

- ½ TEASPOON fine sea salt

- ¼ TEASPOON freshly ground pepper

- 1/3 CUP cilantro leaves, firmly packed finely chopped

- 2 TABLESPOONS mint leaves chopped

- Paprika for garnish

Instructions

1. Place garbanzo beans, water, lemon juice, cumin, coriander, garlic, salt, and pepper in a food processor fitted with a metal blade.

2. Process until smooth and creamy, adding more water as needed to achieve desired consistency.

3. Add cilantro and mint.

4. Pulse briefly to incorporate; herbs should "speckle" the mixture rather than turn it completely green.

5. Spoon hummus into a serving bowl. Sprinkle with paprika before serving.

Ornish Spinach, Apple and Fennel Salad

Preparation time

15 minutes

INGREDIENTS

For Vinaigrette:

• 4 TABLESPOONS apple cider vinegar preferably raw, unfiltered, organic

• ½ TEASPOON orange zest

• 1 TABLESPOON fresh orange juice

• 1 ½ TEASPOONS pure maple syrup

- 1 TEASPOON whole grain mustard

- ½ TEASPOON ground fennel seeds

- ½ TEASPOON curry powder

- ¼ TEASPOON freshly ground pepper

- ¼ TEASPOON fine sea salt

For Salad:

8 CUPS baby spinach

1. 2 apples cored and thinly sliced such as Braeburn, Honeycrisp, or Pink Lady

2. 1 medium sized fresh fennel bulb, about 8 oz cored and thinly sliced (2 cups)

3. 1/3 CUP dry roasted soy nuts (see Chef's Note)

4. ¼ CUP scallions chopped

Instructions

1. To make the vinaigrette, in a small bowl, whisk together apple cider vinegar, orange zest, orange juice, maple syrup, grainy mustard, ground fennel, curry powder, salt, and pepper. Set aside.

2. In a large bowl, toss the spinach with the apples, fennel, soy nuts, and scallions.

3. Season lightly with additional salt and pepper, if desired.

4. Toss with three-quarters of the vinaigrette.

5. Taste for seasoning. Add remaining vinaigrette as necessary. Serve immediately.

Pumpkin Pie

Preparation time

35 minutes

Ingredients

FOR CRUST:

- 9 OZ (ABOUT 14) lowfat graham crackers approved Reversal brand, such as Nabisco low fat

- ⅓ CUP PLUS 1 TABLESPOON unsweetened soy, oat or flax milk

FOR FILLING:

- 1/2 CUP (ABOUT 6 DATES, OR 3 OZ) pitted medjool dates

- 1 1/2 CUPS unsweetened soy, oat, or flax milk

- 2 TABLESPOONS agar agar (sea vegetable flakes)

- ONE 15-OZ CAN unsweetened pumpkin puree

- 3 TABLESPOONS flax meal

- 1 1/2 TEASPOONS cinnamon

- 1 TEASPOON vanilla extract

- 1 TEASPOON ground ginger

- 1/8 TEASPOON ground cloves

- 1/2 TEASPOON fine sea salt

Instructions

1. Preheat oven to 325ºF. To make the crust, crumble graham crackers into the bowl of a food processor fitted with the metal blade. Pulse until crackers form fine crumbs. Add soy milk and pulse until mixture holds its form when pressed.

2. Using your fingers, press the mixture evenly over the bottom and sides of a 9-inch pie pan. Place the pan in the oven and bake until crust is lightly browned, about 10 to 12 minutes. Remove from oven and set on a rack to cool.

3. To make the filling, place dates in a small bowl with 1/2 cup hot water. Cover bowl and let sit until dates are softened, about 10 minutes. Strain, reserving 1/4 cup of the date-soaking liquid.

4. In a medium-sized, heavy-bottomed saucepan over medium heat, combine nondairy milk and agar agar. Bring to a simmer, whisking frequently. Reduce heat and cook, whisking frequently, until agar agar is completely dissolved, about 5 minutes.

5. Remove from heat. Whisk in softened dates, reserved 1/4 cup of date-soaking liquid, pumpkin, flax meal, cinnamon, vanilla, ginger, cloves, and salt. Working in batches if necessary, pour pumpkin mixture into a blender, being careful to fill blender no more than two-thirds full. On low speed, blend mixture until smooth.

6. Pour filling into prepared crust. (You may not need all the filling. Pour any extra into a ramekin or serving dish. Chill and serve as pumpkin

custard.) Place pie in refrigerator and chill for several hours before serving. Pie will firm up and set as it cools. If you like your pumpkin pie served warm, cover the chilled pie with aluminum foil and warm in a 300ºF oven for 10 minutes.

Healthy Pizza Pasta Salad

Preparation time

30 minutes

INGREDIENTS

- 16 oz gluten-free pasta (2 8-oz boxes)

- 1 15-oz can chickpeas or cannellini beans, rinsed and drained

- 1 15-oz can kidney beans, rinsed and drained

- 1 large green bell pepper (or 2 small), seeded and diced

- 1 c julienned sun-dried tomatoes, lightly packed (see note)

- ½ c pitted black olives, sliced

- ⅔ c fat-free or lite Italian dressing (DIY version here)

- 2 tsp dried oregano leaves

- ¼ c toasted pine nuts (omit to keep McDougall-friendly)

Instructions

1. Cook pasta according to directions on package.

2. While pasta is cooking, toss remaining ingredients in a large bowl, reserving 1 Tbsp of pine nuts.

3. When pasta is cooked, rinse with cold water and immediately add to salad. Toss gently to coat.

4. Top with remaining 1 Tbsp pine nuts.

Banana Rice Pudding

Preparation time

1 hour

INGREDIENTS

1. 1 1/2 c Brown rice; cooked

2. 1 md Banana; cut in slices

3. 1/2 ts Ground nutmeg

4. 1 cn Fruit; (15-ounce can), cut in slices

5. 1/4 c Water

6. 1 ts Pure vanilla extract

7. 1 c Nonfat milk

8. 2 tb Honey

9. 1/2 ts Ground cinnamon

INSTRUCTIONS

1. In a medium-size saucepan, combine the banana and fruit slices, water, honey, vanilla, cinnamon and nutmeg.

2. Bring to a boil, reduce the heat, and simmer for 10 minutes, or until quite tender but not mushy.

3. Add the rice and milk and mix thoroughly .

4. Bring to a boil and simmer 10 more minutes.

5. Serve warm.

Lentil Soup

Preparation time

1 hour

Ingredients

- 1 pound lentils

- 1 bay leaf

- 3 large carrots, peeled and sliced

- 2 stalks celery, chopped

- 1 large onion, chopped

- 1/2 teaspoon cumin powder

- 2 cups crushed tomatoes (fresh or canned)

- 2 tablespoons extra-virgin olive oil

- Salt and pepper to taste

- Vinegar (red wine, cider or balsamic, optional)

Instructions

1. Pick over lentils to remove any stones, dirt, or other foreign objects.

2. Rinse them well in cold water and place in a large pot with enough cold water to cover lentils by 6 inches. Add the bay leaf.

3. Bring to a boil, skim off foam, lower heat, and boil gently, partially covered, until lentils are just tooth-tender, 20-30 minutes.

4. Add carrots, celery, cumin and onion to the lentils. Cook partially covered till carrots are tender, about 20-30 minutes.

5. Add crushed tomatoes, olive oil, and salt and pepper to taste. Simmer, partially covered, until lentils become very creamy and soft. Stir occasionally and add boiling water if necessary to prevent sticking.

6. Remove bay leaf before serving. If you like, stir in a little vinegar just before serving.

Black Bean and Corn Salad

Preparation time

15 minutes

Ingredients

- 2 cans of black beans, drained and rinsed well (or 3 cups cooked)

- 1 can fire roasted, diced tomatoes 15 oz

- 1 package of frozen corn, 16 oz., thawed by running under warm water in drainer

- 1/2 purple onion, diced

- 1 can of water chestnuts, drained and rinsed 8 oz

- bunch cilantro, chopped (1/4 cup or more)

- 2 Tbsp lime juice

- zest from 1 lime

- 3 + Tbsps. balsamic vinegar, to suite your taste

• Salt and garlic powder, to your taste

Instructions

1. If using canned black beans, drain and rinse them before using them. To do this, I pour them into a colander and rinse under warm water.

2. Next, place the frozen corn in the colander and run the kernels under warm water to defrost. There is no need to cook it.

3. Dice the purple onion and chop up the cilantro.

4. For the lime, I recommend using a citrus zester to zest it before squeezing out the juice for this recipe. When it's whole, it is much more firm and easy to zest.

5. Combine all ingredients in a large bowl and mix well. The recipe calls for 3 tablespoons of balsamic vinegar, but I love balsamic and actually use a little more.

6. Stir together thoroughly and serve.

7. This tastes even better after a few hours (or next day) after marinating in the refrigerator.